Keto Diet, Don't Harm Yourself

How To Avoid TOP 5 Mistakes on Ketogenic Diet. Keto Guide For Beginners, Includes Meal Plan For Weight Loss, Cookbook and Recipes, Body Healing Plan, Improving Metabolism and Nutrition Facts + Bonus Chapters

© Copyright 2017 - All rights reserved.

The following eBook is reproduced below with the goal of providing information that is as accurate and reliable as possible. Regardless, purchasing this eBook can be seen as consent to the fact that both the publisher and the author of this book are in no way experts on the topics discussed within and that any recommendations or suggestions that are made herein are for entertainment purposes only. Professionals should be consulted as needed prior to undertaking any of the action endorsed herein.

This declaration is deemed fair and valid by both the American Bar Association and the Committee of Publishers Association and is legally binding throughout the United States.

Furthermore, the transmission, duplication or reproduction of any of the following work including specific information will be considered an illegal act irrespective of if it is done electronically or in print. This extends to creating a secondary or tertiary copy of the work or a recorded copy and is only allowed with express written consent of the Publisher. All additional right reserved.

The information in the following pages is broadly considered to be a truthful and accurate account of facts and as such any inattention, use or misuse of the information in question by the reader will render any resulting actions solely under their purview. There are no scenarios in which the publisher or the original author of this work can be in any fashion deemed liable for any hardship or damages that may befall them after undertaking information described herein.

Additionally, the information in the following pages is intended only for informational purposes and should thus be thought of as universal. As befitting its nature, it is presented without assurance regarding its prolonged validity or interim quality. Trademarks that are mentioned are done without written consent and can in no way be considered an endorsement from the trademark holder.

WAIT...

Before You Continue, Grab Your Free Bonus of 3 Low Carb Reports (Value $37) NOW!

I want You to be more prepared for Keto Low Carb lifestyle, that's why I decided to provide you a valuable free bonus straight away. Also, in this way I want to thank you for choosing my book, so simply scan QR code to grab your 3 reports right now!

- KETO AT THE GYM REPORT -
- LOW CARB FAQ REPORT
- 35 TIPS TO GO LOW CARB WHEN EATING OUT REPORT

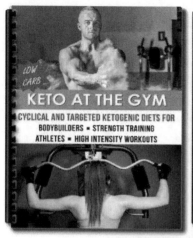
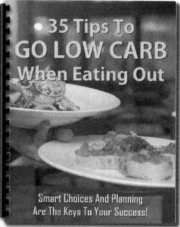
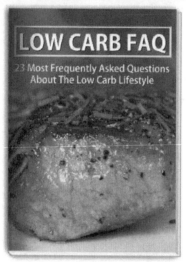

Scan QR code bellow to get FREE BONUS

Table of Contents

Introduction 6

Chapter 1: Keto for Beginners (and Possible Consequences) 7

Chapter 2: Top 5 Keto Mistakes (and How to Avoid Them!) .. 28

Chapter 3: Keto Meal Plan (with Recipes) 34

Chapter 4: Body Healing (How Keto can Help You!) 55

Conclusion 58

BONUS Chapter 1: Low carb diet Q&A 61

Bonus Chapter 2: 147 Low Carb Foods Shopping Lists 64

Bonus Chapter 3: Keto Diet Checklist 70

Appendix 1: Conversion table 75

Introduction

Congratulations on downloading *Keto Diet, Don't Harm Yourself* and thank you for doing so.

The following chapters will discuss everything that you need to know about the ketogenic diet, as well as steps that you can take to avoid harming yourself while you're on it. This book is also going to cover some of the biggest mistakes that people new to keto make and how to avoid making those same mistakes. We'll talk about the *realities* of keto. Everybody always wants to talk about how keto is some savior of a meal plan that is going to cause you to lose a tremendous amount of weight with very little work. While this is partially true, keto is just like any other diet. It has its set of problems that you'll run into as well as a set of "best practices" that you should follow in order to get the most out of the diet.

Now, there is a slight separation between the ketogenic diet and other diets. While other diets can very much be considered "fads", the ketogenic diet is grounded in very sound science. It's been used for a long time for both rapid weight loss in morbidly obese patients as well as to control severe seizures. It's a medically safe diet and the science behind it can make you lose a lot of weight and ultimately change your life. We'll go more into that in the first chapter.

However, it is not a miracle diet. It's going to take work and careful attention and, like any other major lifestyle change, you're going to have to be extremely careful about what you're putting in your body.

There are plenty of books on this subject on the market, thanks again for choosing this one! Every effort was made to ensure it is full of as much useful information as possible, please enjoy!

Chapter 1: Keto for Beginners (and Possible Consequences)

So you've made it this far and by now you're probably wondering what exactly keto *is*. After all, there are mentions of the diet pretty much everywhere. Even celebrities have started to espouse the numerous virtues of the ketogenic diet.

LeBron James turned to a ketogenic version of the Paleo diet in order to lose some weight; Gwyneth Paltrow is releasing a low-carb cookbook called *It's All Good!* and tries to avoid giving her kids carbohydrates, and even Kim Kardashian used a low-carb diet similar to keto in order to shed around sixty pounds of baby weight. So what are they all trying to get at, here?

The ketogenic diet is pretty easy to understand at its core. The thing that makes it different from Paleo is that Paleo's focus is on eating solely unprocessed food, but Paleo permits natural sugars like honey and high-sugar fruits. Meanwhile, keto focuses on restricting carbs. The thing which sets Keto apart from Atkins is that Atkins *starts off* with a ketogenic diet (called the induction phase) which then morphs into something else, adding back in carbs and aiming for a "sustainable" diet.

Keto is based on some essential scientific components that can be a little dense though. Let's start at the beginning.

First off, as you may or may not know, there are three primary components to food known as *macronutrients*. These are *fat*, *protein*, and *carbohydrates*, and all of them are important in their own way in the context of the body's function. For example, fat lubricates the bloodstream and reinforces cell structure. Protein provides essential muscle structure and keeps you strong. Carbohydrates serve the primary function of giving the body energy and spurring essential operations.

The ketogenic diet is based on the idea of *ketones*. The science of ketones is based on the notion that your body needs a source of energy, so it's going to generate energy one way or another. Carbohydrates create an incredibly direct form of energy, but unfortunately, they also come with their shares of side effects. These include burning extremely quickly (leaving you hungry), unprecedented weight retention when you eat too much, and the famous carb crashes when you overeat, lending itself to unstable energy levels. The body, however, is completely aware of how to create a source of energy from another macronutrient: fat. Ketones are the natural result of the body lacking carbohydrates and instead turning to fat as a secondary energy source. This means that your body essentially goes into fat-burning mode and you begin to melt pounds off.

There are numerous other benefits to eating ketogenically, as well. Since fats burn far slower than carbs do, you tend to feel a lot less hungry a lot less often. When you do eat, you won't get the "too full" feeling and you won't feel sluggish or tired after eating anymore either. All in all, the entire way you eat and the entire way you look at food will be changed. Instead of seeing it as a risk-reward thing where you eat but worry about losing weight or eating too much of the wrong kind of thing, food instead becomes a sort of fuel that you use to keep your body. Instead of "emergency" eating (eating when you feel hungry and potentially overeating as a result), you'll feel less hungry and have a different understanding of calories and intake, so you'll instead be eating for the purpose of maintenance. In other words, your entire relationship with food is going to change just by eating on the ketogenic diet.

If this sounds good to you, then you're in luck. This diet won't be easy, but this book is going to cover a lot of the essential information that you need to practice the ketogenic diet safely and melt the pounds away.

So we've established by now that eating on the ketogenic diet entails ketones. How does one generate ketones? Well, essentially, you have to reset the way by which your body creates energy. You can do this simply by changing your eating habits. Your body will almost always burn carbs. However, if there are no carbs to burn, it will naturally switch over to the alternative.

What does this mean for you? Well, it essentially means that switching over to the ketogenic diet is as easy as simply cutting out the carbs out from your diet and replacing those calories with fat.

Now, there are two components to weight loss using keto. The first is to be in *ketosis*, which is the name for the state where your body is using ketones for energy instead of carbohydrates; the second is to actually apply weight loss principles in order to get the most out of your ketosis. We're going to cover these one at a time.

Component one: Entering ketosis

Ketosis is pretty easy to enter into. As I said before, all that you have to do is cut carbs out of your diet and you should be set. What can be hard for somebody who isn't used to paying attention to carbs is that these can sometimes be a little difficult to recognize. For this reason, we're going to take a moment to pay some special and direct attention to what is a carb and what, conversely, isn't a carb.

First off, carbs are pretty much everywhere, so learning to avoid them can be really tough. However, once you learn what foods are okay to eat and what foods aren't, you'll feel a lot more comfortable going forward with your ketogenic diet and won't be checking back with guides and references all of the time.

Remember, the goal here is to enter ketosis. You can enter into ketosis by having less than 50 grams of carbs, for most people. However, it will be a long and strenuous process if you push the upper bounds. On the other hand, you can have your body producing and burning ketones for energy in almost no time at all by simply eating less than 20 grams of carbs per day. You could even push it to 25 grams per carbs and still experience really rapid ketosis. However, it's best to avoid as many carbs as possible and get the majority of your carbs from leafy greens, so try to avoid pushing the boundaries too much as it may make it harder to make a complete transition to the ketogenic lifestyle.

So when you're considering foods that are acceptable to eat, you first have to consider carb content. What are carbohydrates?

Carbohydrates generally present themselves as sugars or starches. In the end, carbohydrates encompass every single thing that will break down and become glucose in the blood. They also encompass a few other things such as dietary fiber and sugar alcohols, primarily because they don't fit other classifications and have similar chemical structures to carbohydrates. These carbohydrates, however, aren't taken into account and are subtracted from the entire carb count. So, for example, natural peanut butter has six total grams of carbohydrates. However, two grams of this exists as dietary fiber. This means that to get the carb count which will impact your blood glucose, you can simply subtract the extraneous carbs (dietary fiber, sugar alcohols, and so forth) from the total carbohydrates. Six minus two leads us four, giving us a total of four *net carbs*. Net carbs can be defined as the carbohydrates which will ultimately have an impact on blood glucose. The goal of entering ketosis is to have less than twenty grams of net carbs per day.

So, knowing that carbohydrates generally present themselves as sugars and starches, you probably have a half-decent idea of where they may start to manifest. Obviously, foods that have added sugars - like cakes, cookies, and brownies - are going to be rather high in carbs. You can add to those foods such as that are clearly starchy like potatoes or taro. However, a lot of people don't take into account that these aren't the only major sources of carbohydrates. Bread is incredibly starchy. So are, for example, rice and pasta. These are major sources of carbohydrates and, for most people, are where the vast majority of their carbohydrates come from.

So obviously when you're starting out on keto, you're going to want to avoid things with added sugars or significant amounts of starches. This means cutting out things like potatoes and bread. You can do so slowly (as we'll talk about in a bit) or all at once.

However, there are more sugars you may not be taking into account. Consider fruit, for example. The sugar in fruits comes primarily from something called *fructose*, which is a major carbohydrate. This doesn't mean that you can't have any fruit at all, but you do need to be rather careful about eating them and do some research. The fruits that are lowest in sugars are going to be the ones you're letting yourself eat. These are generally berries, like blueberries. A little research can go a long way in determining what fruits are alright to eat. You may, however, want to avoid eating fruit altogether, as it may cause you to have bad carb cravings.

You're also going to want to avoid lentils. Lentils can include a variety of foods but generally encompass beans, such as pinto beans, black beans, and green beans. These are a major source of carbohydrates and can add up quite quickly.

So now that you know what *not* to eat, the question still exists of what one *can* eat. This question is actually a fair bit harder to answer. In short, everything that doesn't feature carbs is what you can eat. Anything that keeps you below your designated carb limit is fine for you to eat.

However, this does leave quite a few questions to be asked. So what I'm going to do is go through every major food group and delineate what you can and can't eat on keto:

Meats

Meats are keto's bread and butter. They're chock full of protein and fat, meaning they will absolutely fill you up on energy and keep you going for a long, long while. Most meats also have absolutely no carbs (or very very few) meaning that you can have as much as you would like. A good portion of your keto eating will be meat. This is one of the reasons that keto is fun: you're commonly told to stay away from meat and not eat too much, and also to avoid red meat. You get to throw both of these pieces of advice out the window while you're on keto. It can be a really liberating experience and could be just what you need if you want to eat keto.

Do, however, avoid cured meats such as ham. Cured meats are often brimming with sugars. You can cure your own meat and control how they're cured, if you so desire, which allows you to ensure that there are no extra sugars going into your meat.

Also, while it's not expressly a meat, this is the most fitting category to put it in since it's a direct animal product: eggs. The importance of eggs in a keto diet cannot be understated. When you're trying to eat keto, you're going to want to eat eggs all the time. They'll become a fundamental part of your eating habits! They have no carbs, are very versatile, are full of protein, and are rather tasty to boot. You can use them in sweet dishes, savory dishes, baking, frying, as a binder, as a side, all on their own, as an omelet, poached, scrambled, with extra ingredients or without. Really, eggs are a keto wonder food. They aren't super high in calories but they will most likely become a very important part of your breakfast routine.

Dairy

Dairy is a lot harder to pin down than meats because unlike meats, you can't just have whatever you like.

Let me start by saying that cheese is a foundational part of the ketogenic diet. Cheese has almost no sugars (generally less than 1 gram of carbs per serving) meaning you can have as much as you'd like. It's also rather filling and a great source of both fat and protein. Cheese, then, can be used to spice up vegetables, to pair with meats, or even to have on its own.

If you're going to get some sort of prepared cheese, such as ricotta, be sure that you check the labels. Generally, more organic cheeses will still have rather low carb counts. For example, the difference between supermarket ricotta and organic ricotta can be as many as 10 grams of carbs per serving. Again, take the time to read the label and look at the total carbohydrates. You should be fine as long as you take that precaution.

Milk has *lactose* in it, which is converted into glucose. For this reason, milk explicitly should be avoided. as the carbs add up more quickly than is justifiable. However, milk *products* don't necessarily have to be avoided. An unsugared yogurt - or better yet, an unsugared Greek yogurt - can be relatively low in carbs and provide a great snack. Heavy cream is an important cornerstone of a lot of low-carb cooking and you'll probably be using it rather extensively. Half-and-half has an extremely low carb ratio per serving and you can use it freely as you normally would.

In general, avoid milk. You can replace it really easily with unsweetened coconut or almond milk. Many people actually prefer those, anyway. If you're ever unsure about a dairy product, just read the label and make the judgment for yourself - it's there for a reason!

Nuts

There's quite a bit of variance in the different kinds of nuts. In general, nuts are a fine snack on keto - and arguably one of the better ones - because they are relatively low in carbs, are full of healthy fats, and can be quite filling. However, it's worth noting that some nuts are far higher in carbs than others. Pecans and brazil nuts are among the best, coming in at only 4 grams of net carbs per 100 grams of nuts. Macadamia nuts are slightly higher, coming in at 5 grams, and peanuts and hazelnuts come in at 7 grams. On the other end, however, are pistachios at 18 grams of net carbs per 100 grams and cashews at 27 grams of net carbs per 100 grams. It's a very important distinction to make if you're going to be regularly snacking on nuts.

However, it can't be understated how great of a keto snack these actually are. They're very filling and satisfying treats that will allow you to feel full off of next to nothing. Nuts are a great staple of a good keto diet.

Vegetables

Vegetable consumption can get a little iffy on the keto diet, and it can be hard to tell exactly which vegetables you can and can't eat. There is a general rule you can follow of only eating green and leafy vegetables, but this can also leave the palate a little bored. Your mouth deserves a little bit more nuance than that. As a result, I'm going to go into more detail.

You can actually break down ketogenic vegetable consumption into three categories: *eat often, eat sparingly,* and *don't eat. Don't eat* are vegetables that you should avoid at all cost, *eat sparingly* are vegetables that you can use in other dishes but should never have as a dish themselves and should never have very often, and *eat often* are vegetables that you need to make a staple in your diet. It's very important that you eat vegetables with every meal because it allows you to take in all of their valuable nutrients. And believe me, you're going to want to make sure that you're getting plenty of nutrients.

Vegetables that you should *eat often* are leafy greens in general. These are vegetables such as spinach, lettuce, kale, and broccoli. However, some looks can also be deceiving. For example, cauliflower is an incredible vegetable to eat on keto because it's very low in carbs - even lower than broccoli, for example - and has such a neutral taste that it can be used in pretty much anything. Mushrooms would also fall in this category. Mushrooms are generally very low in carbs and can be used both as flavorings and main courses. You can also use them to accent things like keto burgers, grilling a large mushroom to use as a bun. Avocados are another amazing keto food, extremely filling and full of fat. You can make regular use of those and get a lot of mileage out of them, since they're delicious and leave you full. Also consider zucchini, which you can you can use in things such as zucchini fries or cut up in order to use as a pasta replacement. If you like zucchini, you can even make things like zucchini chips! Hot peppers, such as jalapenos, are also fantastic keto foods. Pickles (and kimchi) are fantastic snacks on keto and can be used pretty much freely. Be wary of the sodium content when using preserved foods, though.

Vegetables that you should *eat sparingly* are those that you can use to accent a meal but should rarely have on their own. In other words, massively limit your consumption of these, because the carbs will most certainly add up. However, that doesn't mean that it's not worth it to get them. They can be an excellent palate cleanser and can be fantastic at adding some variance to your meals. The first which comes to mind are onions. Onions can be a great addition to a lot of dishes and add quite a bit of flavor, but you need to be sparing with them because the carbs in them add up very quickly. There's a reason caramelized onions are a thing - onions are full of sugar in large enough quantities. Sweet peppers, such as bell peppers, are also rather high in carbs. They, in conjunction with onions, add a great foundation for a lot of dishes (such as Italian cooking and Tex-Mex) but can add up rather fast. Feel free to eat them, but be wary of how much you're using and do research. Garlic is fine for you to eat, while on the subject. Tomatoes are another excellent vegetable in this category. They can be refreshing to many and are quite tasty in their own right. They aren't super high in carbs but they still should be used sparingly because it's hard to gauge your servings and overeat and have too many carbs when it comes to tomato. Just be careful, essentially. Carrots also fall into this category. One large carrot has roughly 5 grams of carbs. If you cut it up and steam it or use it in stir-fry, it can add some valuable flavor! However, they aren't for snacking on their own.

Vegetables that you should avoid at all cost are generally the starchy roots. Avoid potatoes, for example, because they have a ton of carbohydrates. Sweet potatoes also fall into this category. So do beets, rutabagas, and turnips. In general, if a vegetable isn't a leafy-green and grows below ground, you probably shouldn't eat it. This may seem a little terse but it's really all that you need to know in this category.

Fruits

Fruits are excellent at satisfying a sweet tooth, especially when you're having bad keto carb cravings. However, they can also exacerbate those same carb cravings, so they're something you need to be wary of. Additionally, the carbs can add up really quickly and fruit generally doesn't have a high enough fiber content to leave you feeling content after a serving. Therefore, you should probably limit your fruit intake in general or just cut it out completely.

When you do eat keto fruit, you'll be astounded at how small the servings are and how many carbs are in each. For example, a half cup of blueberries - which is one of the lowest carb fruits - has roughly 15 grams of carbs. That's an absurd amount! They add up stupidly fast when you're trying to eat a low-carb diet, so avoid them in general as much as you can.

Fats

There's one very good reason that keto is a fun diet, and that's because the old wisdom of limiting your fat intake becomes pretty much invalid when you're eating on it. You can start to shirk that general advice and start instead to eat fats as much as you'd like. This can be really liberating and help push you along even when you can't have carbs. Fats are generally very savory and, well, frankly they make things taste good. That's a biological function because fats have the highest amount of calories, so we're engineered to think that they're the tastiest.

You should in general stick to the "healthier" fats, but always take naturally obtained fats or fats obtained otherwise. Avoid processed fats, too. For example, take grass-fed butter over vegetable oil whenever possible.

There are many fats that you'll start to become acquainted with. Many keto recipes, for example, call for coconut oil because it's a relatively neutral fat that still has a pleasant and subtle taste. You can also drizzle fats as much as you like without worrying about their content. You can garnish your fake pasta with as much olive oil as you like or add some bacon fat to your eggs for more flavor. Really, the choice is up to you. Keto is a low-carb high-fat diet, so you're going to be eating more than enough fats.

Spices and condiments

Spices are generally carbless. However, note that I said *generally*. If a spice is derived from a root of a plant, sometimes it will have higher carbs. Take it from me - I made a keto chicken curry with a ton of ginger without taking all of the carbs of the dish into account. After the ginger, the onion, the curry powder, the coconut milk, the yogurt, and the tomato were all taken into account, I had a dish that was pushing more than 25 grams of carbs, even without the cauliflower bed of rice. It was a shame! I still enjoyed the dish, for certain, but it was hardly what one could call keto.

For the most part, though, you don't have to worry too much about spices. You can add cinnamon and other traditional spices to your heart's content.

When it comes to condiments, things get a little bit more dicey. There are some condiments that are just solutions of vinegar and some kind of base, like mustard (vinegar and mustard seed) or hot sauce (vinegar and chili peppers). These are generally free-reign and you can have as much of them as you would like. When you do get hot sauce, though, read the labels, as some have a lot of added sugar.

For salad dressings, it gets really complicated. The most straightforward dressing you can have is an oil and vinegar dressing. These are really simple. You simply combine your oil of choice (for example, olive oil) and your vinegar of choice (for example, white wine vinegar) in a 3 parts oil to 1 part vinegar ratio, then add salt and pepper to taste and whisk it all together. These have no carbs and a lot of flavors, so you'll get a lot of mileage out of these.

Blue cheese dressings also have a rather low amount of carbs, so you can eat them without too many issues. The same goes for ranch dressing (plain full-fat; avoid buttermilk and low-fat as they will have higher carb contents). Be wary of your servings with these as the serving size is often smaller than a lot of people actually end up using, which means that your four grams of carbs may end up totaling out to be around 8 or even 12 grams of carbs. However, with that in mind, they can be a great way of spicing up your meal and keeping your taste buds entertained, so don't be afraid to use them occasionally.

Unfortunately, many higher-carb salad dressings are out of the question. For example, thousand island dressing is pretty much a no-go unless you make it for yourself. In general, just check the labels and figure out your net carbs and, additionally, be realistic about your serving sizes.

When it comes to other forms of dressings and condiments, follow the general rule of check the label. A really common one is ketchup. When it comes to ketchup, there are some low sugar alternatives you can try out. These still, of course, use tomatoes as a base so their carb count won't exactly be amicable. However, they can go a long way for you if you're a big ketchup fan and craving it. The same goes for barbecue sauce; while the ones you normally get are full of sugars and other non-keto-friendly ingredients, many companies offer low-sugar or sugar-free alternatives that you can try instead. Note that for both ketchup and barbecue sauce, you can also make your own rather easily.

When it comes to condiments and sauces, it's rather easy to figure out what's acceptable and what's not. All that you have to do is read the label and use some common sense. Note that many sauces will have relatively easy keto-friendly versions you can make which are sugar-free and easy on your new diet.

Alcohol

Alcohol can be a bit of a cluster on keto and it can be hard to figure out whether it's acceptable or not. The general line of logic is that alcohol *is* acceptable. However, the liver processes alcohol before anything else, so whenever you drink, your body will stop burning fat while it tries to process the alcohol that you ingested. This isn't too terrible, but if you drink often it could lead to weight gain or stalling of weight loss. Try to save it for special occasions and bad days, or at least reduce a number of times you drink per week to one or two.

So what alcoholic beverages are acceptable on keto? The bottom line is that generally, hard liquors without sugar added or any sort of sugary syrups are your friend. For example, whiskey, spiced rum, and tequila are absolutely fine. However, cinnamon whiskey - which is made by taking whiskey and adding a cinnamon syrup to it - is *not* fine.

In the same vein, many beers have hops or sugar added to them to increase the flavor, both of which obviously will make your favorite beer not very keto. Especially light beers are your best option. Look for beers that specifically advertise their low carb content. These may not be the *tastiest* beers in the world, but they will get the job done and let you kick back and relax for a bit.

Wines are rather difficult, too. Avoid dessert wines at all costs because they have sugar added. The drier the wine, generally, the more acceptable of a drink it is on keto. However, even super-dry white wines can have around 6 to 7 grams of carbs per serving, so keep it light.

Alcohol can be hard to find data for since they aren't legally required to put nutritional information on the sides of alcohol bottles. However, with a little searching, you can often find all of the relevant information you need on various alcoholic beverages.

Starting out on Keto

So now that we've talked about what you can eat, we have to talk a bit about the various ways to get into keto. Now, this book includes a meal plan that you can shop for and then start to work with directly. If you do so, you'll be jumping right in. However, you can also ease in. I'll discuss the difference between the two in just a second.

Before we make that distinction, there's another distinction to be made: *strict* keto versus *lazy* keto. They're both perfectly valid ways to practice the diet and they both have their benefits and drawbacks, too. Strict keto is the method of keto wherein you keep careful tabs on all of your macronutrients and carefully log every single meal that you take so as to stay under a calorie deficit. Lazy keto is where you simply eat less than 20 grams of carbs per day without keeping track of the rest.

Strict keto is the best for weight loss, while lazy keto is the best for long-term sustainability. Strict keto can be a great experience and will almost certainly cause you to lost vast amounts of weight in very little time at all as long as you keep up with it and maintain the diet. Lazy keto is also perfectly fine for weight loss once you become decent at estimating calories. Some people, too, simply lose weight when they do keto; that's how it worked for me! Despite not keeping up with my calories, I still somehow would always lose weight on keto - completely regardless of how strict I was about it.

Personally, I'd recommend newcomers to ease into strict keto. The best way to start keto is to follow the meal plan laid out in this book while you become accustomed to the ketogenic diet, then start practicing strict keto. After a week or two following the meal plan. At that point, you'll be aware enough of what you can and can't eat under keto that you can intelligently make your own decisions about what you're putting in your body.

You can, of course, try lazy keto - especially if you aren't trying to lose weight incredibly rapidly. It may be considerably easier for you in the end if this is the case, and it makes keto into far more of a lifestyle change than a diet. It's very important, too, that you do recognize keto as a lifestyle change rather than a diet because that allows you to start thinking about it in different terms than you normally would. It makes the transition to a long-term change easy which you will very much need. Weight loss isn't something that happens in a day, and if you don't take the time to change your relationship with food entirely, then any weight loss isn't going to end up being kept off, anyway. You have to change the way that you think about food, or else the changes that you make will be pretty much impermanent and you're bound to gain weight back.

Weight Loss Principles

Earlier, I said that there were two components to actually losing weight and making a lifestyle change on the ketogenic, diet: there is the aspect of going *into* ketosis, and there's the aspect of applying *weight loss principles* from there in order to lose weight.

Now, this isn't necessarily set in stone. As I said, not everybody necessarily *needs* to start counting calories in order to lose weight on keto. Some people are going to be successful with it anyway because everybody's body is different.

However, for the vast majority of people, weight loss - whether it's on keto or on some other diet entirely - is going to come on different terms. These terms are that weight loss is a simple process, based upon the concept of *calories in* versus *calories out*. If you take in more calories than you're putting out, then you're going to gain weight; conversely, if you take in fewer calories than you're putting out, then you're going to lose weight. It's a relatively simple concept, but you'd be surprised how many people are adamant that there's a lot more to the equation. The simple fact is that there's not. I've helped a lot of people to lose weight, and so often, people will give me bizarre excuses: *it's not in my genetics to lose weight, my body doesn't work like that*, or any one of myriad strange and, frankly, untrue assumptions about the process of weight loss.

The truth is that it comes down to a really simple equation. If calories in are less than calories out, you lose weight.

This can seem a little intimidating at first, but the truth is that it's not at all. Everybody's body expends *thousands* of calories simply by virtue of the person *existing and breathing.* That's right, this means that technically, you don't even have to work out or be active to lose weight. There's a good chance that your body burns anywhere from 1500 to 2000 calories per day without you putting any work in at all. These are calories which go to run the body's essential functions, like breathing, using your brain, and carrying out internal bodily functions like converting food and oxygen into sources of energy.

So when it comes down to it, you don't have anything to worry about. All you have to do is focus on getting your level of calories below this magical number.

So then you have to ask, "how do I determine this magical number?" Well, this magical number has a name, first off: your *basal metabolic rate*, or *BMR*. This is frequently referred to as your "metabolism", though there are without a doubt better titles for this phenomenon. This number is based on a few different things, those being your height, weight, and age. This all play an important part in determining your metabolic rate. Somebody who is older is going to have a slower metabolism than somebody who is younger; somebody who is taller or heavier is going to naturally take up more energy than somebody who is shorter or skinnier.

At this point, you probably want to make the decision as to whether or not you'd like to take on lazy keto or strict keto. If you're just trying to lose weight over a longer period of time, lazy keto is significantly easier to pick up and start doing than strict keto is, where there's a bit of a learning curve.

If you're planning to do strict keto, then you need to download MyFitnessPal. The handy thing about MyFitnessPal is that it will automatically configure your MBR based off of the information that you enter when you sign up for a profile. You can configure all of your settings and basically start from there. Strict keto isn't particularly difficult but it is quite a bit of stress. Using MyFitnessPal helps you to mitigate this stress and pretty much make it a non-factor, though, so long as you're willing to keep careful track of your meals. You can configure your specific macronutrients by setting your specific diet plans. The general percentages for somebody eating on the ketogenic diet are that 70% to 75% of the diet will be composed of fat, while 20% - 25% of the diet will be composed of protein and 5% will be composed of carbs. These numbers can vary depending upon your personal dietary choices, but these are the general line for keto.

If you're planning to do lazy keto, however, you're going to want to just calculate your BMR. There are several resources for this that you can Google in order to find - unfortunately, links don't go over well in eBooks. Once you've calculated your MBR, all you have to do is eat less than twenty grams of carbs per day. Pay close attention to labels and mentally try to calculate how many calories you take in each day. You can estimate, of course; it's called lazy keto for a reason! The only caveat with lazy keto is that your weight loss may be slower than it would be otherwise.

With that, you're set up to carry out weight loss principles under ketosis and start losing weight. Remember - it's a simple game of calories in and out! One thing to understand about weight loss is that diet is the number one factor in weight gain and weight loss. If you were to run a mile, you would only burn about 100 calories - which is roughly equivalent to a teaspoon of peanut butter. The truth is that almost all of weight loss happens through adjusting your diet.

So with all of that out of the way, the question stands: what exactly *will* your weight loss progress look like? Well, you should see a *lot* of weight melt off your first week. This is because your body is depleting its glycogen stores and you are losing a lot of water weight. It's not uncommon for people to drop around five to ten pounds of water weight in their first week.

The rest is ultimately up to you. The weight loss rate on keto compared to other diets, for most people at least, can be up to twice as fast. So in the time that you'd lose a pound on a normal low-fat high-carb diet, you may lose twice as much in the same amount of time. This, of course, is conjecture and highly personal. At any rate, you will almost certainly lose weight on the keto diet, and do so with extreme ease.

Once you're on keto, you may be wondering what exactly you should expect. Well, it will vary. First off, you should expect the keto flu. Being ill-prepared for the keto flu is the number one mistake that most people make, and we'll talk about it at length in the next chapter. However, most people feel rather ill for their first week or two in while their body adjusts to using ketones instead of carbohydrates. There's a good reason for this, but as I said, it'll be explained in-depth in the next chapter.

Another thing that you should expect is that you'll need to drink a *lot* of water. Ketosis has diuretic properties, meaning that it's going to make you pee rather often. You're going to have to replace the lost water as much as you can in order to preserve your body's natural balances and keep yourself from becoming dehydrated. This can't be understated.

Aside from those, you may have brain fog initially as a result of keto, but most people find that this goes away very soon.

This is contrasted by several benefits later on. For example, many people find that once they're adjusted to keto, they will find that they have a far clearer way of thinking. They also find that they are rarely hungry as a result of the fact that the body is burning fats instead of carbs. They find that they have much greater endurance when working out because of the slow burn of carbs as well, and don't experience the energy bursts that happen with carbs. In other words, carbs are better for burst energy while fats are better for extended energy. This also naturally goes in hand with the fact that on keto you will no longer be sluggish or tired after a big meal because your body doesn't burn fats like it does carbs.

Many people find that they far prefer the way keto makes them feel to the way a "normal" diet feels, which makes it rather easy for them to stick with it over a long period of time. Your mileage may vary, of course; some people simply don't like the way that keto makes them feel. This is alright too. The only way you're going to know is by trying it out, though. There are no major observed health problems that can arise from trying a low-carb diet, so it is most certainly worth your time to give it a shot.

In the end, keto can be a fantastic vehicle for weight loss. It's not particularly *easy* to understand and get into, but it can be a really fulfilling lifestyle change and can easily land you with the body that you'd like to have. In the next chapter, we're going to discuss some of the biggest mistakes that many people make on the ketogenic diet - and how you can avoid them.

Chapter 2: Top 5 Keto Mistakes (and How to Avoid Them!)

The ketogenic diet is no different from any other major medical change in that it can be quite easy to rough yourself up if you do it the wrong way. Luckily, there are some things that you can do in order to make your time on keto far more enjoyable and also mitigate any potential health consequences that could arise. We're going to go through these one by one and discuss all of their finer points so that you can be properly prepared.

Mistake #1: Not Being Prepared for Keto Flu

The keto flu is one of the worst parts of keto. When you are friends with people who *aren't* doing keto and they want to go out to eat, they'll often ask - "why can't you have a cheat meal? The food here is pretty healthy!". With you being new to keto, you yourself may not even understand the answer to this question. Well, the short answer is that the keto flu is not fun at all. It feels like you've got a flu, along with all of the fogginess, nausea, and lethargy that comes along with that.

Many people have figured out how to beat or altogether avoid the keto flu, though. There are no major health consequences to the keto flu and it will resolve itself over time, but it's still not fun at all to deal with, so naturally it's best to figure out how to avoid "contracting" the keto flu in the first place, or at least mitigating its effects when it does come around.

In order to understand how to avoid and beat the keto flu, you have to understand what it is and why it happens. When you start to go into ketosis, your body undergoes a lot of changes.

The most immediate is that you start getting rid of stored sugars through urination. However, this also comes with the finer point that when you urinate, your electrolytes are also released. The keto flu is the unique end result of combining the dehydration which occurs during this period with the electrolyte imbalance that many people fall victim to.

So what can you do about it? Well, there are a few things. The first is an age-old remedy, and it works on the same basis that people with the *real* flu drink soup: broth is *fantastic* for restoring your electrolyte levels and getting both fluids and sodium at the same time. Grab any sort of stock you like (or bouillon cubes) and have them on hand, ready to prepare, so that when you start to feel the keto flu coming on, you can make some. You could even make it as a preventative measure: make a cup of broth in the morning and before bed (as well as throughout the day if necessary) from the moment you start keto, which will help you to be ready to take on the keto flu and perhaps avoid it altogether. It will certainly lessen the symptoms when they do crop up.

What else can you do? Well, apply more salt to things and also consider picking up Lite Salt. Lite Salt is a combination of potassium and sodium which still offers a salty taste but will let you get some potassium as well. Apply it liberally to any food for a perkier and fuller taste and to ensure you're getting potassium.

When it comes to magnesium, make sure you're eating leafy greens as part of your keto diet. Spinach and other leafy greens - and *especially* raw okra, if you like raw okra - can be a fantastic source of magnesium and potassium both, so be sure that you're eating these. Artichokes are particularly high in sodium, but be certain that you're eating French/Globe artichokes and not Jerusalem artichokes, as Jerusalem artichokes are high in carbs, totaling around ten grams of carbs for the entire vegetable.

Another way to resist the keto flu is by making sure that you're taking in plenty of water. Taking in water is essential to keeping your body running and keeping yourself, well, hydrated - which is especially important at a time when you're peeing out a lot of your electrolytes.

Mistake #2: Not Exercising

This one is a big deal. It's really easy to pick up keto and just start losing weight on it, sure, and as I said earlier on in the book, the biggest component of weight loss is that you take in fewer calories than you put out and that generally, all comes down to diet.

However, it's not the *only* factor. The fact is that when you're losing weight, you need to find some time to work out if at all possible or at least keep active. This is just for the sake of your general health. The biggest thing that you can do for your health is starting to exercise. Even though you may lose weight, your body still isn't in "shape". When you exercise, it increases the amount of work your heart can do and makes it even stronger, as well as makes you feel better in general. Being in shape is extremely important, and simply losing weight will *not* get you there.

Mistake #3: Trying to Lose Too Much Too Fast

It's really easy to try to lose more than 2 pounds per week and dial on huge calorie deficits with the idea that you're going to "fight through the pain". However, even 2 pounds per week can really be too much. The body isn't prepared for drastic changes in any way, and this is an easy way to send your body into a "shock" state. It can take a toll on your overall health and can lead to you being far weaker and losing important muscle mass.

What's more is that if you ever find yourself eating less than 1,000 calories per day, you're probably eating too few. For most people, 800 is the starvation threshold. Your body is not made to function on that few calories.

Additionally, if you try to lose a ton of weight all at once, your body is *not* going to look good. You are going to develop a lot of loose skin and you will not be in proper shape. You may look better than you did when you were fat, but by just practicing proper patience, you can slim down *and* look good. The only excuse for rapid weight loss is if you're already heavy enough for it to be a major strain on your health, and even then, there's no excuse for eating less than 1,000 calories per day ever. Don't do that. You will hurt yourself.

In the end, I'm sure you've heard that phrase before that weight loss is a marathon and not a sprint. Take your time. If you try to eat too little, you may end up burning out and hardly losing any weight at all. Take it easy on yourself and just try to lose 1 to 1 and a half pounds per week. Most nutritionists recommend losing no more than 1 pound per week, but I lost 2 per week without any major consequences. Just be careful going forward that you aren't losing weight *too* rapidly. Losing more than 2 pounds per week almost certainly isn't healthy.

Mistake #4: Eating Too Much Salt/Processed Food

It's really easy to get lazy on keto just because you don't want to make food and pre-prepared keto food can be rather expensive. It can then be *extremely* easy to just buy things like Vienna sausages, SPAM, and hot dogs because they're all keto friendly and just eat those whenever you're hungry.

Not so fast, though. If you eat too much processed food, you may quickly find that you're taking in *too much* sodium. This - especially in combination with having too much caffeine regularly - can contribute to higher blood pressure. Mine got dangerously high because, at one point, my meals were mostly processed food. I caught on and started taking care of it prior to that, but it's still not something you want to play chance with.

Avoid a possible tragedy by taking pains to make sure that you aren't taking in *too much* sodium. Early in on keto, you're going to want to take in a lot, but still, there's a certain point where you can eat *far* too much and you want to definitely try to avoid that mark.

Mistake #5: Not Eating Enough Vegetables

This one is huge. When you're doing keto, fat packs so many calories that you can pretty much subsist off of meat and cheese if you really want to. However, this will come back to haunt you later. You need to make certain that you're eating enough vegetables.

While a normal diet has numerous different sources that common vitamins and minerals may come from, like fruit, bread, and various related foodstuffs, the keto diet is generally devoid of these aside from leafy greens. Leafy greens are also full of dietary fiber which will keep your body running smoothly in a time where you're already putting it under a lot of stress.

As a result, the best thing that you can do for yourself on keto is to make sure that around half of your plate, every meal, is composed of low-carb vegetables - or at least to the greatest extent that you can! If you do this, then you can guarantee that you'll be getting all of the nutrients that your body needs in order for you to feel comfortable, happy, and healthy.

Keto can be rather difficult to adjust to, and there are some grave mistakes that you can make while you're on it. With that in mind though, through concentrated effort, you can avoid some of the biggest mistakes and keep yourself healthy. Keto is a perfectly safe and healthy diet as long as you're doing it the right way. You do it the right way by eating fresh foods and keeping as much of an eye as you can on essential things such as your electrolytes.

(Enjoying this book so far? I'd love to see your review on Amazon. Please, scan QR code to leave a review. Thank you!)

Chapter 3: Keto Meal Plan (with Recipes)

This chapter is going to focus on setting you up with seven days worth of meals so that you can hit the ground running with the ketogenic diet! Pick one from each category every day for a week. Enjoy!

Southwest omelet
Eggs and bacon
Keto pancakes
Keto oatmeal (ricotta)
Scrambled eggs and avocado
Bulletproof Coffee

Caprese salad
Chicken salad
Chicken lunch wrap
Jalapeño Poppers
Keto tuna salad
Keto deviled eggs
Keto Thai coconut soup

Keto nacho bake
Keto stir fry
keto curry
Keto burger with mushroom bun
Avocado Feta mix
Meatza
Loaded cauliflower

Breakfast

Southwest Omelet

Ingredients:
- 3 eggs
- Jalapenos, chopped
- Cheddar cheese (or fiesta blend)
- Bacon, cooked and chopped
- Onion, chopped
- Hot sauce
- Cilantro
- Sour cream

1. Beat the eggs then put them in a skillet over medium high heat.
2. Let cook, then add other ingredients one by one.
3. Fold over then cook on either side for a minute.
4. All done! Enjoy it. Garnish with fresh cilantro and enjoy with fresh avocado.

Eggs and Bacon

Ingredients:
- 3 eggs
- Bacon

1. Cook eggs how you like them. Pan fry bacon. Serve and enjoy!

(This may seem really straightforward, but not every keto breakfast has to be flashy. This one *is* straightforward, and that's part of its allure. You don't have to spend a long time working on it. You can get it done in 10 minutes, eat, and be out the door.)

Keto Pancakes

It's easy to miss pancakes when you're on keto. They're tasty and delicious - how could you not? Fortunately, this recipe has your back.

Ingredients:
- 2 ounces of cream cheese
- 2 eggs
- Cinnamon
- Sugar-free maple syrup
- Sucralose (Splenda) powder

1. Combine cream cheese, eggs, cinnamon, and a little Splenda in the blender.
2. Blend up and then start cooking on the oiled skillet over medium heat until they're golden brown like pancakes. Take off.
3. Then run Splenda through the blender until super fine.

This is "powdered sugar". Top finished product with your powdered Splenda and sugar-free maple syrup. Voilà! A delicious breakfast that's super easy to make.

Keto Oatmeal

This may not sound very good, but it is, trust me. Look for the highest quality ricotta that you can get. Organic ricotta can have as little as 2 grams of net carbs while store-brand ricotta generally has *at least* 7 grams of net carbs. Again, be wary and always read labels to find the best option.

- 0.5c of ricotta cheese
- Cinnamon
- 2 tablespoons butter
- Splenda

Combine ingredients, then microwave together. Mix and enjoy. It takes all of 2 minutes to make, but it tastes absolutely delicious and extremely filling!

Greek Eggs

Ingredients:
- Feta (to taste)
- 3 eggs
- ½ cup spinach
- Avocado, chopped and spritzed with lime juice
- Oregano or Greek seasoning
- Salt and pepper to taste

1. Scramble eggs then remove from heat.
2. Add in feta, spinach, and seasoning, then put back over low heat, stirring often for about 2 minutes.
3. Remove from heat and stir in fresh avocado. Add salt and pepper to taste.

Bulletproof Coffee

Here's the thing: this isn't *exactly* Bulletproof Coffee. Bulletproof Coffee is made from MCT oil, which is a derivative of coconut oil. However, this will let you give it a try and decide if you like it or not. Many people who do keto take Bulletproof Coffee as their breakfast option since it's fatty, tasty, and takes no time to make.

- Hot coffee
- 2 tbsp coconut oil
- 2 tbsp grass-fed organic unsalted butter (Kerrygold is fantastic for this!)

1. Combine ingredients in blender and blend. Enjoy!

Lunch

All of the lunch selections in this book are meant to be enjoyed cold, meaning you don't even have to reheat them. Just prepare them and store them in the fridge, then grab them on your way to work the next day!

Caprese Salad

This salad is super easy to make *and* is delicious. Get the highest quality mozzarella and olive oil that you can, because they make or break the taste. This is best enjoyed when tomatoes are in season.

Ingredients:
- Basil
- Fresh mozzarella
- Tomato
- Olive oil

1. Slice mozzarella and tomato. Arrange in a repeating pattern with basil - basil, mozzarella, tomato - then top with some olive oil. You're all done! Enjoy it!

Chicken Salad

Ingredients:
- Roasted or grilled chicken
- Rosemary
- Romaine lettuce
- Cherry tomatoes
- Mozzarella cheese, shredded
- Spinach
- Roasted almonds
- Olive oil
- White wine vinegar
- Salt/pepper

1. Combine all ingredients aside from oil and vinegar.
2. Toss and store.
3. Then combine 1 part vinegar to 3 parts oil and mix with salt and pepper.
4. Garnish salad with oil and vinegar dressing when ready to eat.

Turkey Lunch Wrap

Ingredients:
- Low carb tortilla
- Turkey (shredded or carved as lunch meat)
- Colby jack cheese
- Tomato
- Lettuce
- Onion, sliced
- Spinach
- Cucumber, sliced

Combine all ingredients in low carb tortilla (can be found in store next to normal tortillas) then wrap up and store.

Jalapeño Poppers

Ingredients:
- 5 jalapeños
- 5 strips bacon
- 8oz cream cheese
- 1 packet of ranch dressing mix

1. Preheat oven to 350 degrees.
2. Melt cream cheese and mix with ranch dressing blend.
3. Cut jalapeños in half, then remove core and seeds.
4. Cut bacon strips in half.
5. Spread cream cheese mixture on inside of jalapeño halves.
6. Wrap each jalapeño half in a bacon half.
7. Bake for 15 minutes.

All done! Having this cold will still be delicious but will take some of the edges off. You can also reheat. Enjoy with full-fat low-carb ranch dressing.

Keto Tuna Salad

Ingredients:
- 2 cans of tuna, drained
- Dried onion flakes to taste, one to two teaspoons is good
- Salt and pepper
- Boiled egg, chopped
- 1 tbsp sour cream
- ¼ cup of mayonnaise
- Dash of dill

No instructions necessary. Combine all ingredients and you're ready to go!

Keto Deviled Eggs

Ingredients:
- ¼ cup of mayo
- a touch of mustard
- 1 tbsp of chives
- 1 bsp of bacon bits
- Salt and pepper
- 6 eggs, boiled

1. Halve your boiled eggs and take out the yolks. Mash separately.
2. Combine all ingredients with mashed yolks, then put this mixture in each of the boiled egg whites.
3. Store until ready to eat.

Keto Thai Coconut Soup

Ingredients:

Broth

- 1 quart of broth
- 2 cups of coconut milk
- Lime zest
- ½ tbsp of lemongrass, dried
- Sliced jalapeño
- Thumb of ginger, sliced
- 1tsp sea salt

Soup

- 3.5 ounces of shrimp
- 1 tablespoon coconut oil
- 1 ounce of sliced onion
- 1 ounce of sliced mushroom
- 1 tablespoon fish sauce
- lime juice
- Cilantro for the garnish

1. Put all broth ingredients together and simmer for 15 minutes.
2. Strain, then simmer again, then throw in your shrimp and fish sauce.
3. Add the soup vegetables, then simmer until the shrimps are tender.
4. Add your lime juice then serve with your cilantro garnish.

Dinner

Keto Nacho Bake

Ingredients:
- Ground beef
- Onion, chopped
- Bell pepper, chopped
- Jalapeño, chopped
- Tomato, chopped
- Fiesta blend cheese
- Sour cream
- Cilantro

1. Preheat oven to 375 degrees.
2. In a cast-iron skillet, brown the ground beef. Once it has been browned, drain off any excess fat - not necessary!
3. Add in chopped vegetables and stir up until well-blended.
4. Top with thick layer of fiesta blend cheese then pop in the oven. Bake until cheese is melted.
5. Remove skillet, then top with cilantro. Serve with sour cream.

Keto Stir Fry

Ingredients:
- Onion, sliced
- Thumb of ginger, chopped
- Bell pepper, sliced
- Pork, cooked and cut into bite size pieces
- Broccoli
- One carrot, sliced
- Soy sauce

1. Sauté ginger, onion, and bell pepper together until onions are browned.
2. Add in broccoli and carrot and put a lid over ingredients, allowing to steam.
3. After everything has steamed, add in your pork and soy sauce. Replace lid and cook for 10 more minutes over low heat.

Keto Curry

Ingredients:
- 2 chicken breasts, cut into bite size pieces
- Sliced red pepper
- Bean sprouts
- 1c coconut milk
- Mushrooms, chopped
- 3 zucchinis cut into strips
- Red curry paste
- Onion, sliced
- Clove of garlic, minced
- Red pepper, sliced
- Cilantro

1. Sauté onions and chicken until chicken is almost finished.
2. Add everything else aside from coconut milk and red curry paste.
3. Add coconut milk and 3 tbsp of red curry paste, then cook over medium heat. Add seasonings as desired.
4. When it boils, everything is done. Garnish with cilantro.

Keto Burger with Mushroom Bun

In my opinion, good burgers are best done with just ground beef and seasoning, but some like to add an egg as a binder. Do so if you want.

Ingredients:
- Ground beef, fattest available
- Salt, pepper, garlic powder, coriander
- Cheddar cheese
- Portabella mushroom
- Burger condiments as desired

1. Combine ground beef and seasonings. Cook all the way through. Allow cheese to melt on patty as burger finishes.
2. While burgers cook, slather olive oil on your mushrooms (remove the stem first) and then toast in a separate skillet.
3. Place finished burgers in mushroom cap and then add your condiments. Top with another mushroom cap to have fully prepared burger.

Greek Guac

Ingredients:
- Avocado
- Feta (to taste)
- Onion, chopped
- Clove of garlic, minced
- Tomato, chopped
- Lime juice
- ½ cup spinach, chopped
- Salt and pepper, heavy

1. Combine ingredients and salt heavily. Eat straight or with celery strips.

Meatza

Ingredients:
- Ground beef
- 2 eggs
- Low-carb pizza sauce
- Shredded mozzarella
- Italian seasoning
- Olive oil
- Pizza toppings as desired

1. Preheat oven to 375 degrees.
2. Combine ground beef and eggs, adding salt and pepper if desired.
3. Grease pizza pan with olive oil, then put ground beef in pan, spreading and evening as much as possible, keeping it cohesive so there are few cracks (the cracks will widen during cooking).
4. This is the "crust". Throw it in the oven and cook until it's browned, about 20 minutes.
5. Remove it, then turn the oven heat up to 425 degrees.
6. Put your pizza sauce on the crust, then your mozzarella. Top with pepperoni or sausage or whatever takes your fancy, really. Finish off with an olive oil garnish and Italian seasoning.
7. Throw your meatza in the oven for 5 minutes - long enough for the cheese to melt.
8. Take it out and enjoy!

Loaded Cauliflower

Ingredients:
- 1 head of cauliflower
- 1c shredded cheddar
- 3 slices bacon, cooked and chopped
- Butter
- 2 tbsp chives, chopped
- Sour cream

1. Break cauliflower apart into florets. Run through a food processed until it has the consistency of rice. Then add a bit of water and microwave, covered, for five minutes. This will steam it.
2. Add chives, seasoning, and half of the cheese. Mix.
3. Top it with leftover cheese and bacon. Broil for a minute or two.
4. Enjoy hot, add your butter and sour cream when serving.

Chapter 4: Body Healing (How Keto can Help You!)

Keto has for quite a long time been used for its medical properties. For example, it first came into popular use as a treatment for epilepsy. However, there are many cases where the ketogenic diet has been shown to help in many more ways than just this.

For example, the ketogenic diet has been proven to assist in both the stabilization of mood and the regulation of hormones. This can go a long way for your day-to-day life and your day-in/day-out mental health. Stability in all senses is important, and the ketogenic diet will allow you to bolster that stability.

It also has been shown to improve both one's memory and one's cognitive processing. These are beneficial for obvious reasons and will help one to improve their day to day life, being more wakeful and momentous.

Ketosis has been shown time and time again to reduce the signs of aging when followed over the long term. The mechanisms behind this aren't entirely obvious, but they are there, one way or another.

Ketosis is often used in the management of Alzheimer's disease and cancer both, with numerous indications of improvement in the latter.

Additionally, being in ketosis has fantastic anti-inflammatory properties. Due to the fact that it can massively reduce the amount of cellular inflammation due to a lack of cellular oxidizing. Therefore, if you try to take on keto, you may see a reduction in normal inflammation, if it's something that you deal with on a daily basis.

When you go on keto, your body is in a very diuretic state where it's emptying its glycogen stores. However, alongside this, if you're eating a "proper" keto diet and taking in a lot of fiber as a result, you'll also find that you're getting rid of a lot of toxins as well. This can lead to you feeling better overall since your body is in a far cleaner state.

Also, when you're on keto, your body is far less confused about how it should "spend" energy obtained from food. Processes become a lot less muddied as the body just tries to have each specific nutrient do its job. This means that keto lends itself perfectly to muscle regeneration as protein will be used more effectively. You also are generally taking in more protein than usual on a keto diet which can help quite a bit, as well. While on the note, for the record, there's a lot of division in the keto community about how much protein is *too* much. This is nonsense. The idea is that if you have "too" much protein, the body will undergo a process called gluconeogenesis whereby the body tries to take excess protein and convert it into carbohydrates. There is, however, very little real scientific basis for this. While it does happen, it occurs extremely slowly and not within nearly great enough number to knock you out of ketosis. There's almost no chance that you could consume enough protein in order to knock you out, in fact. You can always err on the side of caution if you'd like, but it's better to get "too much" protein than too little because too little can lead to devastating muscle loss. Allow me to remind you that you're not trying to lose your *lean* body mass!

The bottom line is that keto isn't a miracle diet. However, there are numerous properties of keto that make it a fantastic option for the management of several conditions. Additionally, there are some innate properties of the keto diet and ketosis itself that lend it towards being an excellent way to take care of yourself. There are almost certainly healing properties to ketosis, and these properties are beyond worth your time and energy to explore.

Conclusion

Thank for making it through to the end of *Keto Diet, Don't Harm Yourself*, let's hope it was informative and able to provide you with all of the tools you need to achieve your goals whatever it may be.

The next step is to take the steps forward and start practicing keto. This book has armed you quite well to tackle the ketogenic diet and to know exactly what obstacles and problems you may run into along the way. It's my solemn hope that you're well prepared for any issues which might arise and that you're quite happy and ready to start with the ketogenic diet.

If you ever get confused, there are a whole lot of online resources available that will help you to stay on the safe side when you're doing keto, as well as help you out when you reach inevitable plateaus. The internet provides an amazing foundation for support in anything, and keto is gaining a lot of steam lately in and of itself, so there is absolutely no reason that you shouldn't take full advantage of these opportunities and see what you can do.

In the end, I believe that what you were looking for was an opportunity to learn not only what the ketogenic diet *is*, but also some of the possible downsides of doing it, as well as how to mitigate the chance of running into those problems. I've said it numerous times throughout this book, but keto is not a miracle diet. It is not some magical solution that you can just do and then lose a million pounds overnight. There will be times where you find it particularly challenging, dull, or you feel downright sick. However, even in these harder times, there is a very good reason to keep going: your health. A lot of diets will get you where you need to be, but you're here for a reason: the ketogenic diet is gaining a reputation for being a phenomenal way to lose weight. You owe it to yourself to take that much of a chance, try out this revolutionary diet plan, and become the person that you'd really like to be.

So in that mission, I hope that I've provided you an excellent book that you'll be able to look back on and reference for the future to come as you try to work your way through the ketogenic diet and reach that end goal that you have in mind. If you enjoyed this book and you thought it was a solid and informative read, I'd love it if you'd leave me an Amazon review. Those reviews help me to know exactly what I'm doing right and wrong so that I can keep producing quality content.

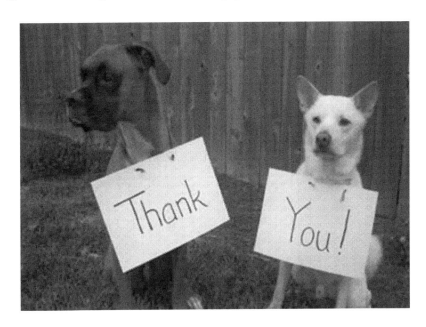

(Please, scan QR code to leave a review on amazon. Thank you)

Good luck in your ketogenic journey, and I wish you well!

Oh, wait...

I hope You didn't forget your FREE BONUS - Instant Access to 3 Low Carb Reports.

- KETO AT THE GYM REPORT -
- LOW CARB FAQ REPORT
- 35 TIPS TO GO LOW CARB WHEN EATING OUT REPORT

Scan QR code bellow to get FREE BONUS

BONUS Chapter 1: Low carb diet Q&A

WHAT IS A LOW CARB DIET?
A diet that is very low in carbs where carbs are replaced with healthy fats and their reduction triggers a metabolic state known as ketosis where the body uses fat instead of dietary carbs for energy.

WHAT CAN I EAT?
Meats/Protein: Turkey, chicken, red meat, ham, sausage, bacon, organ meat and exotic fowl. Fish, seafood and eggs. *Produce*: all non-starchy vegetables and possibly a little berries. *Fats*: grass fed butter, extra virgin olive oil, coconut oil, avocado oil and whole avocados. *Dairy*: heavy cream, full fat sour cream, salad dressings and full fat cheeses in moderation. *Nuts*: almonds, walnuts, peanuts, nut butters, sunflower seeds, and flaxseed in moderation. *Others*: salt, herbs and spices, low carb sauces.

WHAT CARBS ARE NOT ALLOWED?
All refined sugar, sweets, fruit, rice, pasta, bread, grains, starchy vegetables and beans. A slow integration of some carb rich foods, like nuts, berries, and beans takes place in the later phases of the diet and how much you can have depends on individual weight monitoring and the carb's effects on ongoing weight loss and management.

HOW MANY CARBS CAN I EAT?
This depends on the particular plan, the strictest recommendation is 20 grams or less daily, as with the Ketogenic Diet and Atkins Lifestyle. Overall, 50 grams or less daily is recommended.

HOW CAN IT BE HEALTHY TO CUT OUT CARBS FROM MY DIET?

Non-starchy vegetables are allowed and they are the healthiest carbs, it is the unhealthy carbs that are cut out, like refined sugar along with grains, like rice and pasta, including whole grains, which are not much different from sugar, have a higher glycemic index than sugar, lack the nutrients or longevity of fats and proteins, and have been strongly associated with autoimmune diseases. The healthy fats provide essential nutrients, energy and promote the fat burning process, ketosis.

ISN'T LOW CARB JUST ANOTHER FAD?

Absolutely not, it is a lifestyle change, and is not something intended as a temporary fix or a quick weight loss scheme.

WHAT ARE THE HEALTH BENEFITS OF A LOW CARB DIET?

Weight loss, appetite control, prevention and management of diabetes, reduction in visceral fat, stable blood sugars, healthy blood pressure, and may lower risks for heart disease, cancer, and stroke. Used to treat some cancers, traumatic brain injury, epilepsy, Parkinson's disease, Alzheimer's disease and polycystic ovary syndrome.

DO I HAVE TO COUNT CALORIES?

Low carb diets advocate eating to satisfaction, and not counting calories. When you eliminate unhealthy carbs, you also get rid of out of control cravings, stabilize blood sugar and consequently the appetite, and research has shown that reducing carbohydrates and replacing them with protein and healthy fats results in reducing overall caloric intake naturally and without starvation.

HOW WILL MY BODY RUN IF I CUT CARBOHYDRATES? AREN'T THEY WHAT FUEL US?

Yes, carbohydrates are a source of fuel but they are not the only ones, evidence shows that our bodies run better when burning fat as opposed to carbs, a process known as ketosis, which is triggered by eliminating insulin trigger carbs.

There is also a natural process in the body that turns protein into glycogen fuel called gluconeogenesis. So you will have plenty of fuel, better health and weight loss.

Bonus Chapter 2:
147 Low Carb Foods Shopping Lists

MEAT, FISH AND POULTRY
Zero Carb Foods
All Red Meat
Chicken
Turkey
Pork
Veal
Lamb
Fowl (duck, goose, hen, quail)
Organ Meats (tongue brains, liver, heart, and kidneys)
Game Meats (ostrich, venison, caribou, bison, and elk)
Exotic Meats (such as ostrich and emu)
Cold Cuts And Ham (read label some have added sugar)
Bacon
All Fish

SEAFOOD
Shrimp – 0 Carbs
Crawfish - 0 Carbs
Crab - 0 Carbs
Lobster – 2 grams per 6 ounces
Mussels – 8.4 per 6 ounces
Oysters – 12.4 per 6 ounces
Scallops – 3.9 per 6 ounces
Clams – 8.7 grams per 6 ounces
Squid – 7 grams per 6 ounces

FATS AND DRESSINGS
Butter - 0 Carbs
Mayonnaise - 0 Carbs
All Oils (plant oils are best: olive, avocado, coconut, sunflower, soy, sesame) - 0 Carbs
Pure unrefined cold pressed extra virgin coconut oil (Contains Medium Chain Triglycerides fatty acids, metabolized by the body to be used as immediate energy and not stored as fat) - 0 Carbs
Avocados – 4.8 grams each
Blue Cheese Dressing (2 tbsp.) – 2.3 grams
Italian Dressing (2 tbsp.) – 3 grams
Cesar Dressing (2 tbsp.) - .5 grams
Ranch Dressing (2 tbsp.) – 1.4 grams
100 Island Dressing (2 tbsp.) – 4.8 grams

SOY VEGAN PROTEIN
Soybeans - 6.2 grams per 1/2 cup
Soy Milk – 1.2 grams per cup
Firm Tofu – 2.2 grams per 4 ounces
Silken Tofu – 3.2 grams per 4 ounces
Tempeh – 16 grams per cup
Soy Nuts – 2 grams per ½ ounce

VEGETABLES
Alfalfa Sprouts - .4 grams per cup
Daikon – 1 gram per ½ cup
Endive - >1 gram per ounce
Escarole - >1 gram per ounce
Arugula - .2 grams per ½ cup
Bok Choy - .8 grams per 1 cup/raw
Celery - .8 grams per 1 stalk
Chicory Greens - .6 grams per ½ cup
Green Onions - .1 per 1 tablespoon

Cucumber - 1 gram per ½ cup sliced
Fennel - 3.6 grams per 1 cup
Iceberg Lettuce - .1 grams per 1/2 cup
Jicama - 2.5 grams per ½ cup
Parsley - >1 gram per ounce
Bell Peppers - 2.3 grams per ½ cup
Radicchio - .7 grams per ½ cup
Radishes - .9 grams per 10 pieces
Romaine Lettuce - .2 grams per ½ cup
Artichoke (1/4 Steamed) – 4 grams
Artichoke Hearts In Water - 2 grams per 1 heart
Asparagus - 2.4 grams per 6 spears
Bamboo Shoots - 1.1 grams per 1 cup
Broccoli - 1 gram per 1/2 cup
Brussels sprouts - 2.4 grams per ¼ cup
Cabbage - 2 grams per ½ cup
Cauliflower - 2 grams per 1 cup
Chard - 1.8 grams per ½ cup
Collard Greens - 4.2 grams per 1/2 cup
Eggplant - 1.8 grams per ½ cup
Hearts of Palm - .7 grams per 1 heart
Kale - 2.4 grams per ½ cup
Mushrooms – 1 gram per ½ cup
Kohlrabi - 4.6 grams per ½ cup
Leeks - 1.7 grams per ¼ cup
Okra - 2.4 grams per ½ cup
Black Olives (10 small, 5 large, or 3 jumbo olives) - 1 gram
Onions - 2.8 grams per ¼ cup
Pumpkin - 2.4 grams per ¼ cup
Sauerkraut - 1.2 grams per ½ cup
Spinach - .2 grams per ½ cup
Summer Squash - 2 grams per ½ cup
Tomato (1 medium) - 4 grams
Cherry Tomatoes - 4 grams per cup
Turnips - 2.2 grams per ½ cup

FRUITS
Limes – 2 grams per 1 ounce
Lemons – 2 grams per 1 ounce
Rhubarb - 1.7 grams per ½ cup
Apricots – 5 grams per fruit
Strawberries – 11 grams per cup
Blackberries - 7 grams per cup
Raspberries – 5 grams per cup
Red Grapefruit - 9 grams per 1/2 fruit

DAIRY
Egg White – .3 grams
Egg Yolk - .3 grams
Whole Egg - .6 grams
Heavy Whipping Cream - .5 to .7 grams per tablespoon
Half-and-Half - .5 to 1 grams per tablespoon
Plain Full Fat Greek Yogurt - 9 grams per cup
Full Fat Sour Cream - 2 grams per 4 tablespoons
Unsweetened Almond Milk – Less than 1 gram per cup

CHEESES
Gruyère Cheese - .1 grams per 1 ounce
Cheddar - .5 gram per ounce
Fontina - .4 grams per 1 ounce
Havarti - .7 grams per 1 ounce
Parmesan - .9 grams per 1 ounce
Gouda - .6 grams per 1 ounce
Mozzarella - .6 grams per 1 ounce
Ricotta - .8 grams per 1 ounce
Blue Cheese - 1 gram per 1 ounce
Edam - .4 grams per 1 ounce
Monterey - .1 grams per 1 ounce
Muenster - .3 grams per 1 ounce
Provolone - .6 grams per 1 ounce
Neufchatel - .1 to .8 grams per 1 ounce

HERBS AND SPICES
All Herbs And Spices Have Very Few Carbs

NUTS & SEEDS
Almonds (2 tbsp. whole) – 1.4 grams
Peanuts (2 tbsp.) – 1.8 grams
Hazelnuts (2 tbsp. chopped) - 1 gram
Macadamia Nuts (2 tbsp. chopped) -.9 grams
Pecans (2 tbsp. chopped) - .6 grams
Pine Nuts (2 tbsp.) - 1.7 grams
Pistachio Nuts (2 tbsp.) - 3.1 grams
Walnuts (2 tbsp. chopped) - 1.1 grams
Pumpkin Seeds - 5 grams per ounce
Sunflower Seeds (2 tbsp.) – 1.5 grams
Almond Butter - 3 grams per tablespoon
Peanut Butter – 2.4 grams per tablespoon

ZERO CARB DRINKS
Water
Unsweetened Tea
Unsweetened Coffee
Club Soda
Diet Soda (be cautious as artificial sweeteners can affect low carb weight loss)
Sugar Free Sparkling Water
No-Calorie Flavored Seltzers
Herbal Tea (without added barley or fruit sugars)

ZERO CARB ALCOHOLIC BEVERAGES
Gin
Rum
Vodka
Whiskey
Martini
Tequila

MISCELLANEOUS

Shirataki Noodles – 0 Carbs
White Vinegar – 0 Carbs
Balsamic Vinegar – 0 Carbs
Red Wine Vinegar – 0 Carbs
Rice Vinegar (seasoned) 3 grams per tbsp.
Soy Sauce - 1 gram per tablespoon
Mustard – 0 Carbs
Unflavored, powdered gelatin (use as a binder in recipes) – 0 Carbs
Most Hot Sauces – 0 Carbs
Turkey or Beef Jerky (not teriyaki flavor) - 3 grams per ounce
Kale Chips - 8-12 grams per ounce
Coconut Flakes - 4 grams per ounce
Pickles - 1 gram per pickle

Bonus Chapter 3: Keto Diet Checklist

CARB INTAKE

- Most of the carbs should come from non-starchy vegetables
- Green, fibrous vegetables are your best choices, though many other low carb vegetables are fine
- Always accompany a carb with either a fat or a protein

NET CARBS

- The Ketogenic diet only counts Net Carbs as fiber content in food decreases the overall carb content's ability to impact blood sugars
- Net Carb Formula: Total Carb Count of a Food Minus Fiber Count

LOTS OF HEALTHY FATS

- In ketosis, fat is the main energy source for the body
- Fats provide satiety, boost metabolism and support the enjoyment of food
- Provide key macronutrient requirements
- Natural fats are fine when reducing carbs
- The best fats are monounsaturated and saturated, including olive oil, grass fed butter, and coconut oil
- Margarine is never advised, as it is fake and interferes with ketosis
- Limit intake of polyunsaturated fats, including soybean oil, corn oil, and cottonseed oil

- Fat intake is variable and depends on weight loss goals
- It is not advisable to eat so much fat that you send your caloric intake through the roof

WHEN IN DOUBT, EAT LESS CARBS AND MORE FAT

- Daily Fat Intake Guidelines
- These will vary by body size
- 2 to 3 eggs
- 1 to 2 tablespoons of butter
- 2 tablespoons of heavy cream
- 2 tablespoons of olive oil when cooking or for salad dressings
- 2 ounces of cheese
- 4 to 6 ounces of meat, chicken, seafood, or fish at each meal
- ½ an avocado or 10 olives
- 1 to 2 ounces of nuts or seeds
- Use canola, peanut and grapeseed oils for pan cooking and stir-frys
- Use full fat mayonnaise, canola oil mayo is a good choice
- 1 tablespoon of coconut oil contains ketosis boosting MCTs (medium chain triglycerides)
- Avoid low fat foods, including reduced fat dairy as they have carbohydrates, and chemical compounds

ADEQUATE PROTEIN

- Protein is both 46% ketogenic and 58% anti-ketogenic, as some protein will convert to glucose in the bloodstream and inhibit ketosis, so intake should be enough to prevent muscle loss, but not so much that will disrupt ketosis.

- General Protein Intake Guidelines
- Sedentary lifestyle: 0.69 - 0.8 grams per pound of lean body mass
- Mildly active: 0.8 to 1 gram per pound of lean body mass
- Heavy strength training/bodybuilding and exercise: 1 to 1.2 grams per pound of lean body mass
- Lean body mass is typically defined as - body weight minus body fat. You can use any of a number of online lean body mass calculators, such as this one - *http://www.calculator.net/lean-body-mass-calculator.html* to figure yours.

Protein Choices

- Fatty red meats
- Chicken with skin
- Turkey
- Eggs
- Deli meats
- Seafood
- Fish
- Pork
- Veal
- Lamb
- Fowl (duck, goose, hen, quail)
- Organ meats (tongue brains, liver, heart, and kidneys)
- Game meats (ostrich, venison, caribou, bison, and elk)
- Eggs
- Nuts, seeds and full fat dairy in moderation as they do contain some carbs

EAT TO SATISFACTION

- Eat when hungry until you feel satisfied, but not stuffed

INCREASE SALT INTAKE

- A little extra salt can help avoid possible side effects as your body adjusts to ketosis, including headaches, muscle cramps, or weakness that occurs as result of an electrolyte imbalance and since a low carb diet is naturally diuretic, you don't have to avoid salt to minimize water retention.
- Get that salt from 1 to 2 cups of broth daily or soy sauce over food
- Caution: ask your doctor about increasing salt, and if you are being treated for a condition that requires limited sodium intake, like hypertension continue with the medical advice of your doctor.

DRINK LOTS OF WATER

- Water is a natural appetite suppressant
- Supports the body's ability to metabolize fat
- Several studies found that reducing intake of water might cause fat deposits to increase, while drinking more reduces them
- Hydration greatly promotes weight loss, so drink lots of fresh water throughout the day
- The more active you are the more hydration you will need

I hope you find this bonus chapters useful. I would love to see your review on Amazon. Please, scan QR code bellow to leave a review on amazon. Thank you and good luck.

(QR code for leaving a review)

And don't forget about your Free Bonus - **Instant Access to 3 Low Carb Reports.**

Scan QR code bellow to get FREE BONUS

Appendix 1: Conversion table

I understand that it might get confusing with measurements when trying to cook something delicious, so for your convenience I've decided to include the Conversion table. I hope this will help you to dive deeper into tasty Keto recipes that are provided in this book. Enjoy!

Oven Temperature Conversions

Fahrenheit	Celsius	Gas Mark
250 F	130 C	1/2
275 F	140 C	1
300 F	150 C	2
325 F	165 C	3
350 F	177 C	4
375 F	190 C	5
400 F	200 C	6
425 F	220 C	7
450 F	230 C	8
475 F	245 C	9
500 F	260 C	10

Liquid Volumes

Imperial (UK)	Metric	U.S.
½ fl oz	15 ml	1 tbsp
1 fl oz	30 ml	1/8 cup
2 fl oz	55 ml	¼ cup
3 fl oz	85 ml	1/3 cup
4 fl oz	115 ml	½ cup
5 fl oz	140 ml	2/ cup
6 fl oz	170 ml	¾ cup
7 fl oz	200 ml	7/8 cup
8 fl oz	230 ml	1 cup
16 fl oz	455 ml	2 cups (1 US pint)
20 fl oz (1 UK pint)	570 ml	2 ½ cups

Weights

Metric	Imperial
15 g	1/ oz
30 g	1 oz
60 g	2 oz
90 g	3 oz
125 g	4 oz
175 g	6 oz
250 g	8 oz
300 g	10 oz
375 g	12 oz
400 g	13 oz
425 g	14 oz
500 g	1 lb
750 g	1 ½ lb
1 kg	2 lb

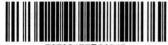

Made in the USA
Columbia, SC
12 October 2017